THE POSTPARTUM DEPRESSION JOURNAL

THE
POSTPARTUM
DEPRESSION
JOURNAL

Prompts and Exercises for
Reflection, Healing, and Self-Care

Rachel Rabinor, LCSW, PMH-C

ROCKRIDGE
PRESS

To my clients past and present, who have trusted me with their most personal struggles and triumphs along their journey to and through parenthood.

For general information on our other products and services or to obtain technical support, please contact our Customer Care Department within the United States at (866) 744-2665, or outside the United States at (510) 253-0500.

Rockridge Press publishes its books in a variety of electronic and print formats. Some content that appears in print may not be available in electronic books, and vice versa.

TRADEMARKS: Rockridge Press and the Rockridge Press logo are trademarks or registered trademarks of Callisto Media Inc. and/or its affiliates, in the United States and other countries, and may not be used without written permission. All other trademarks are the property of their respective owners. Rockridge Press is not associ- ated with any product or vendor mentioned in this book.

Interior and Cover Designer: Jill Lee
Art Producer: Maya Mellenchuk
Editor: Chloe Moffett
Production Manager: Holly Haydash
Production Editor: Melissa Edeburn

Author photo courtesy of Studio Luniste

Paperback ISBN: 978-1-63878-328-2
R0

CONTENTS

INTRODUCTION

The adjustment to parenthood rarely looks like it does in the movies. When I had my first child, I was a therapist working with pregnant and parenting teens. At 30-something, I thought I had it together. I was wrong. My world was shaken, and life never returned to what it once was.

Whether you've been formally diagnosed with postpartum depression or simply feel different than you imagined you would after becoming a parent, you can find support for your perinatal healing and growth in this journal. Perinatal refers to the time before, during, and after childbirth. The perinatal period includes pregnancy through the first—if not the second—postpartum year.

This journal invites you to reflect on your experiences; examine your thoughts, values, hopes, and dreams; and participate in exercises that will help you reconnect with yourself and become the best version of yourself for you and your child.

For more than 20 years, I've supported parents and their children in various capacities. I pursued my master's degree in social work with a passion for reproductive and perinatal mental health brewing in my bones. Life experience and my work taught me how important the mental health of parents is to a child's development.

In 2008 I began working with pregnant and parenting teens. I knew I was in the right place, doing meaningful and powerful work. My own transition to parenthood and reproductive traumas helped refine the future of my career: supporting parents on their journey to and through parenthood.

It's an honor to support my clients, and I'm thrilled to help guide you along your perinatal journey. Identifying your strengths and weaknesses can help you develop strategies to cope with the physical, emotional, and mental strains of parenthood. This journal will assist in this exploration, and I'm hopeful the new skills and tools you learn will support you today and beyond.

This book is not a replacement for seeking treatment for postpartum depression or anxiety. If your symptoms begin to affect your ability to cope with life at home and work or cause serious distress in relationships with others, you should seek treatment from a trained mental health professional. You can find local resources through Postpartum.net, as well as the Resources section on page 146.

Understanding Postpartum Depression

Postpartum depression is one of many perinatal mood and anxiety disorders (PMADs), including perinatal anxiety, perinatal traumatic stress disorder, perinatal obsessive-compulsive disorder, perinatal bipolar disorder, and perinatal psychosis. PMADs are extremely common: 15 to 20 percent of birthing individuals will develop a perinatal mood or anxiety disorder, and 8 to 10 percent of their partners will.

Although they are more prevalent in birthing individuals, it's important to know that pregnancy and a full-term delivery are not requisites for developing a PMAD. Individuals who adopt a child are also susceptible to developing a PMAD, as are those who have miscarried or terminated a pregnancy. Another important fact surrounds the relationship between partners and PMADs: Research shows that when the birthing partner is struggling with a PMAD, the risk to the partner doubles. Getting help when necessary is critical for the health of your entire family.

There are many risk factors for developing a PMAD. Some are biological (nature) and others are environmental (nurture), including:

- Personal or family history of mental illness
- Traumatic pregnancy or birth
- Difficult experiences around pregnancy or birth
- A history of violence or abuse
- A traumatic childhood
- Stress

Although many individuals may feel depressed after having a baby, the most common symptoms are anxiety and overwhelm. Too many people don't reach out for help because they assume that because they aren't depressed, they must not have a PMAD. Other symptoms include the following:

- Feelings of helplessness, hopelessness, or both
- Difficulty in making decisions
- Changes in sleeping and/or eating patterns
- Isolation and withdrawal from community and loved ones
- Frequent feelings of "I can't do this"
- Not feeling like yourself
- Intrusive thoughts, images, or fears of harm coming to your baby that you cannot stop and that you know are wrong
- Irritability, impatience, or rage
- Difficulty concentrating
- Difficulty attaching to and bonding with your baby
- In the most serious cases, seeing, hearing, or feeling things that are not really there, holding beliefs that are not based in reality, or both

You may experience all or some of these symptoms.

Healing Through Journaling

These journal exercises and evidence-based techniques are intended to help you gain greater awareness of your thoughts and feelings while recognizing unhelpful patterns that may be impacting your mental health. I hope you will not only learn new strategies to manage your symptoms and develop greater self-compassion, but you will also shift your mindset to one of hope.

Writing helps you not only process your thoughts, feelings, and emotions, but also manifest your hopes and dreams. Expressive writing is proven to decrease physical and emotional symptoms. Viewing your inner thoughts in the written form allows them to become more concrete and offers an opportunity to learn about yourself and alter your future path.

Please remember to be patient with yourself as you begin this healing journey. Life is very full with a small baby; this transition is likely the biggest one you've gone through as an adult. Although there's no specific amount of time you need to journal each day, consistency will help you improve your symptoms and reach your goals as quickly as possible. It may be helpful to enlist a therapist or a loved one to support you as you do this work. If that's not an option, give yourself permission to move at a pace that feels right for you.

Taking this step toward healing is not easy, but you are worth it. And know you are not alone.

HOW TO USE THIS JOURNAL

This journal comprises three parts covering the physical, mental, and social aspects of postpartum depression. You can start at the beginning and move through it from cover to cover, or pick and choose based on the issues you're struggling with.

Each section of the journal contains three main elements: prompts, practices, and quotes.

- **Prompts** encourage you to reflect and process your experience through writing.
- **Practices** invite you to explore your mind and body through experiential exercises like mindful breathing, visualization, and yoga (don't worry: thorough instructions are included).
- **Quotes** are inspirational or thoughtful words by others to encourage reflection and hope.

This journal is designed to help you experiment with new strategies to grow through this challenging time. Working through this journal will help you discover new coping tools and approaches to manage your emotions today and for the parenting journey that lies ahead. Healthy habits are created one step at a time. Let's get started!

PART 1

Taking Care of Your Body

Most people focus on the emotional or mental aspects of postpartum depression and often ignore the clues our physical bodies provide, even though they are just as prevalent. If you've experienced stomachaches, nausea, headaches, or backaches with no diagnosis, you're not alone. Some new parents experience intense anxiety or panic that feels like a heart attack. Postpartum depression may also show up as fatigue, shifts in appetite, and general exhaustion. These physical manifestations are often overlooked and minimized as part of the normal adjustment, not only by new parents but also by health-care providers.

Trauma is held in the body, often presenting as physical pain and discomfort. Whether you've experienced a recent trauma—infertility, loss, traumatic birth—or have a history of trauma, you may find these events come up as you move through this part of the journal. Please consider additional support from a licensed therapist trained in PMADs and trauma. Resources are available on page 146.

This section explores the effects of PMADs on the physical body and offers methods of self-care and other strategies to help you heal. In addition to the support offered here, it's important to rule out underlying health conditions that may be contributing to your physical symptoms. In addition to traditional Western doctors, I often refer to naturopathic doctors who specialize in uncovering the root cause of symptoms. Please visit Naturopathic.org for local resources.

CONNECTING WITH YOUR BODY

Although the world is full of suffering, it is also full of the overcoming of it.

—Helen Keller

Identifying Your Pain

It's easy to ignore the role your body plays in your overall well-being. However, mindfully tuning into body sensations can open you up to new information. Mindfulness involves paying attention to what is emotionally and physically present.

1. Think back over the past few months and circle any symptoms you have experienced that continue to cause you discomfort.

2. Underline any symptoms you've discussed with a family member or health-care provider.

3. Draw a line through any symptoms you have been dealing with since before your baby arrived.

4. Get curious about your symptoms. If they have lasted longer than two weeks, reach out to your doctor.

   Here are some symptoms people struggling with postpartum depression report.

Fatigue

Sleeplessness

Restlessness

Difficulty falling asleep

Difficulty waking up

Waking in the middle of the night (not because of baby)

Increase in appetite

Decrease in appetite

Difficulty concentrating

Gastrointestinal pain or discomfort

Joint pain

Skin problems

Nausea

Stomach pains

Chest pains

Headaches

Other _____

_____

Share your experience with this exercise and the physical symptoms you've been coping with.

Body Scan

A body scan meditation is a helpful way to release tension you might not realize you're experiencing. Consider using one of the guided body scan meditations available through the UCSD Center for Mindfulness (available on the "guided audio and video" page under the "mindfulness and compassion resources" tab), noted in the Resources section (page 146).

Find a comfortable position, seated or lying down.

1. Allow your eyes to close if comfortable.

2. Take a few breaths. As you do, notice the weight of your body supported by the ground, the sofa, the chair, or wherever you are resting. Feel what it is like to rest your body as you breathe.

3. Bring your attention to the top of your head and scalp. Notice any throbbing, heat, tingling, or strong sensations—or nothing at all.

4. Shift your attention to your face—forehead, nose, jaw, and chin—where tension is often stored. Allow the muscles to soften.

5. On the next out breath, lower your focus to the neck. Let the throat, back, and sides of the neck soften, noticing any sensations that arise on the surface of the skin or deeper within.

6. Continue in this slow, intentional way to scan your body, all the way down to your toes.

7. When you've finished, come back to the journal and reflect on your experience using the prompts over the next few pages.

BODY SCAN REFLECTIONS

Reflect on your experience of completing the body scan practice. What did you notice about your body? Was any area of your body calling for attention? Was any area tense or painful? Did you feel relaxed?

EMOTIONS IN YOUR BODY

Emotions are often connected with certain body areas. A lump in your throat or a pit in your stomach may signal fear. An expansion in your chest may signal pride. What emotions did you notice as you scanned your body? Was there something new?

PHYSICAL PAIN IN YOUR BODY

Do you experience any ache, pain, or tension in specific parts of your body? Keeping in mind emotional and mental tension can cause physical tension, share your reflections about your own physical pain.

IMPACT OF EMOTIONS ON RELATIONSHIPS

The ability to recognize emotional responses in your physical body can affect your relationships with others. Write about a time you lashed out at someone you love and later realized things got heated way too quickly. Identifying physical clues can help slow down the interaction and allow you to respond rather than react.

NAME IT TO TAME IT

When you name your emotions or thoughts, you can tame your physical response, according to Dr. Dan Siegel. Think of a recent time when you reacted instead of responded to someone you care about. What emotion sparked that interaction? Was it anxiety? Fear? Can you identify the part of your body that was sensing that emotion? What do you think that emotion was trying to tell you?

Felt Sense

The felt sense is a term coined by philosopher Eugene Gendlin of the Focusing Institute. It's a combination of emotion, awareness, intuitiveness, and embodiment. This exercise offers an opportunity to gain greater awareness of the felt sense. You will need colored pencils, pens, crayons, or markers. Using the body map, color the areas of your body where you currently sense discomfort, pain, tightness, or tension. Select colors that represent the type of sensation you are feeling in a particular part of the body. Think about the type of pressure and the strokes you use to best reflect the sensations in those parts of the body.

After completing the body map, label the colored areas with emotions. Then write any observations you have about your body map and this process.

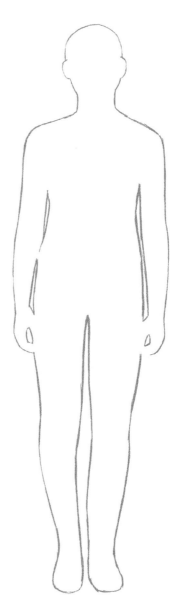

LIFESTYLE INVENTORY

Taking care of yourself is one of the biggest challenges when becoming a new parent. With limited sleep, and feedings 'round the clock, it's not unusual to find yourself skipping meals, sleep, and sometimes even water. Take an inventory of where you are in regard to the following areas of health (think about the quality, quantity, etc.):

Exercise

_____

_____

Sleep

_____

_____

Diet

_____

_____

Relaxation

_____

_____

Spirituality

_____

_____

Smoking

_____

_____

Alcohol

_____

_____

Tobacco

_____

_____

Caffeine

_____

_____

Supplementation with vitamins or other recommended products

_____

_____

Other

_____

_____

_____

IMPROVING YOUR WELL-BEING

What did you learn about yourself after completing the lifestyle inventory? What areas of your health could benefit from change? Choose three areas from the inventory and name one small change that would improve your physical health for each. Reflect on how you would feel if you were to make those slight changes for a week. A month.

Reducing Physical Pain

It's understandable that someone might say, *"Of course your back hurts; you're holding a baby all day."* But it's incredibly frustrating when you feel like your pain is being minimized by friends, family, and even your doctor. Pain can be debilitating and impact your day-to-day living, as well as your mental state.

Here is a list of specialists who can support your physical body before, during, and after pregnancy. Draw a line connecting the specialist on the left with the description of the work they do on the right. Consider the internet search your friend as you complete this activity and learn about the support available to you.

Pelvic floor physical therapist	A. Trained in traditional Chinese medicine. Inserts small needles into your skin at specific locations. Typically helps treat pain, and can also help contribute to overall wellness, including alleviating stress.
Massage therapist	B. Evaluates for restrictions of mobility or movement as well as the cause of pain that may be felt in another connected region of the body.
Chiropractor	C. Focuses on the relationship between the spine and the nervous system, with an emphasis on treating pain by manually adjusting the spine.
Acupuncturist	D. Uses touch to manipulate muscles to relieve pain, help heal injuries, improve circulation, relieve stress, and increase relaxation.
Cranial sacral therapist	E. Diagnoses, prevents, and treats acute and chronic illness to restore and establish optimal health. Works to identify and treat underlying causes of illness, rather than suppressing symptoms.
Naturopathic doctor	F. Uses a light-touch manual therapy to release tensions and restrictions deep in the body in order to relieve pain and dysfunction and improve overall health.

Key: Acupuncturist (A); Pelvic floor physical therapist (B); Chiropractor (C); Massage therapist (D); Naturopathic doctor (E); Cranial sacral therapist (F)

Which specialists will you research to support your healing? Where can you get recommendations for specialists in your community?

SLEEP

There's no way to be a perfect mother and a million ways to be a good one.

—Jill Churchill

SLEEP PATTERNS

Take a moment to think about your relationship with sleep. Is sleep something you cherish or dread? Does the thought of going to sleep bring you comfort or distress?

SLEEP ASSOCIATIONS AND ATTITUDE

Reflect back over the past couple of weeks. When you think about falling asleep, does it bring a sense of relief? Stress? Both? Take a moment and reflect on the attitude you bring to falling asleep.

FALLING ASLEEP

Difficulty falling asleep plagues many of us. Have you had trouble falling asleep since you've become a parent? Did pregnancy alter your ability to fall asleep? Now go further back in time before you were pregnant. Write a few lines sharing what you notice as you reflect on your own pattern of falling asleep during these three stages of your life.

FALLING BACK TO SLEEP

Since becoming a parent, what is it like to be up multiple times in the night? Do you fall back to sleep right away or do you stay awake for long stretches? How do you eventually fall back to sleep?

SLEEP HYGIENE

Sleep hygiene is a fancy way of saying sleep health. What is your bedtime routine like? Do you do the same things to help you return to sleep when you wake up in the middle of the night? What works and what doesn't?

MIDDLE OF THE NIGHT WAKINGS

Shifting into parenting mode from sleep mode requires new parents to adapt quickly. How do you manage middle of the night wakings with your baby? Do you sometimes wake up even if your baby is asleep?

SLEEP AND SCREENS

You've likely heard about the negative impacts of blue light from phones and the recommendation to have a screen-free hour before bed. This sounds good in theory, but many new parents survive middle of the night wakings with the welcome distraction of their phones. What is your relationship with your phone or TV like during the night? Is it a help or a hindrance to sleep?

Progressive Muscle Relaxation

Progressive muscle relaxation can help calm your mind and body by systematically tensing and relaxing specific muscles. As you inhale, you actively tense each muscle group, without straining, for about five seconds. With the exhale, you release the tension and relax the muscle. This exercise can be especially useful for those who feel tension in their body as a result of stress or anxiety. It's also recommended for anyone who has difficulty falling asleep or getting back to sleep.

Feel free to skip any areas where you have pain or discomfort. You can practice this exercise on your own, beginning with your head and slowly moving down your body, but I recommend starting with one of the many audio recordings available so you can truly relax. Once you've practiced with the recordings for a few weeks, it will be easier to do on your own. You will find several recorded options in the Resources section (page 146), or you can search online to find one that's a good fit.

After completing the practice, take a few moments to reflect and share your experience.

YOUR SLEEP PREFERENCES

The average person requires seven to nine hours of sleep to function properly. New parents often get far less, and the impact over time can be debilitating to their physical and mental health. Before you became a parent, how much sleep was your body used to getting? Reflect on how you manage now with less consistent sleep.

YOUR BEDTIME ROUTINE

What does your bedtime routine look like? Are there shifts you can make in your routine—both before getting into bed for the first time as well as during middle of the night wakings—that may help foster healthier sleep? Some examples might include drinking a cup of tea, playing quiet music, dimming the lights, turning off screens 30 to 60 minutes before bed, massaging your feet with lotion, or playing a guided meditation or sleep story using one of the apps listed in the Resources section (page 146). What small changes can you make to help you get more rest?

NOURISHMENT

One cannot think well, love well, sleep well, if one has not dined well.

—Virginia Woolf

ASSESSING YOUR HUNGER

When feeding a new baby around the clock, you can lose touch with your own biological needs. Take a moment to assess your hunger level. How do you feel right now? Are you a bit hungry? Stuffed or too full? Or do you feel content and properly nourished? What sensations are you in touch with? On a hunger scale where 0 is "very hungry" and 10 is "very full," where are you right now?

YOUR APPETITE CHANGES

What and how you eat is related to how you experience appetite and hunger. Have you noticed an increase or decrease in your appetite lately? Take a moment and compare to when you were pregnant and before you were pregnant.

FOOD PREFERENCES

Food choices influence your overall mood and well-being. Have you noticed any changes? Is there any difference in your desire for fruits and vegetables? Sweets? Pasta? Share what you notice when you think about your appetite in these three periods of time: before pregnancy, pregnancy, and postpartum.

FINDING AND MAKING TIME TO EAT

New parents often neglect their own needs for nourishment and food. Recall how you have been eating the last few days. Are there times you have had a rushed meal? A relaxed meal? Forgotten to eat? What do you notice about your eating patterns related to your overall mood?

MOVEMENT

Each morning we are born again. What we do today is what matters most.

—Buddha

Mindful Walking

Mindful walking combines the benefits of mindfulness with the stress-relieving rewards of exercise. If you're unable to get out on your own, bring your baby along. And if you find yourself up walking the halls with your baby at night, try making it a mindful walk!

1. Begin by walking slowly.

2. Notice the beginning of your step, the middle, the end, and the pause between steps before your next foot starts moving.

3. Bring your awareness to your feet. Your awareness will drift to the baby, the mile-long to-do list, the fear that you will never again sleep through the night. Notice these thoughts. Then come back to your feet.

4. Notice your posture. Notice whether your arms are swinging or resting on your baby or the stroller.

5. Notice the sounds and smells around you.

6. Notice what you're seeing.

7. Come back to your feet if your mind begins to drift.

8. Notice the earth beneath you.

Share your reflections on mindful walking.

YOUR DAILY ROUTINE

Becoming a new parent often means your old routines go out the window. Previously, a typical day may have involved multiple errands related to your own schedule. Now it has likely transformed to hours upon hours of holding and feeding your baby. Becoming sedentary can create a strain on you physically and mentally. What was your pre-baby life like? What's the biggest adjustment to your physical body in becoming a parent?

_____

_____

_____

_____

_____

_____

_____

_____

_____

_____

_____

_____

_____

_____

_____

FEELING STUCK

Does exercise just feel like another thing to do? Exercise releases endorphins that have been proven to help reduce stress, decrease anxiety and depression, boost self-esteem, and improve sleep. What kind of exercise have you enjoyed in the past? Spend a few moments visualizing yourself exercising, then share your thoughts.

HEALING

Self-compassion involves treating yourself the way you would treat a friend who is having a hard time.

—Kristin Neff

GETTING OUT IN NATURE

Time in nature is proven to decrease mental distress, increase focus, and enhance happiness, positive social interactions, and a sense of meaning and purpose in life. The latest research recommends spending 120 minutes outdoors in nature per week in any combination of minutes or hours. Does this amount of time seem doable for you? What are some nearby places you can go to spend time outside?

Making a Plan to Connect with Nature

Research shows that mental health improves when you spend time outdoors, whether you're in a forest, by a body of water, or even visiting an urban park. What is your connection to nature? Have you always thrived in nature, or do you choose the city every time? Take a few moments to think and plan an excursion in nature. What support do you need to make it happen?

ASSESSING YOUR SELF-TALK

How do you treat yourself when you're struggling with physical pain or discomfort? When you can't sleep and you haven't been outside in two days or eaten anything green since you can remember, do you take it easy on yourself, offering soothing words of calm? Do you talk harshly to yourself? Share how you most often respond to yourself.

Letter to a Friend or Loved One

Some people struggle with offering themselves tender care and compassion. If that sounds like you, try to put this part of you aside while you participate in this exercise. Imagine your cousin, sibling, or best friend was struggling with physical pain or discomfort like you after becoming a parent. What would you tell them? How would you respond when they tell you they're in pain? Would you tell them to stop complaining or to ignore it? Write a letter to your loved one offering the support you think they deserve.

PRACTICING SELF-COMPASSION

Developing self-compassion is a practice. It doesn't happen overnight and it requires regular effort. Reflect on what you have learned about the way you talk to yourself about your physical discomfort compared with how you would talk to someone you care for.

PART 2

The Path to Emotional Well-Being

Experiencing depression or anxiety after the arrival of a new baby is overwhelming. These feelings can make it difficult to concentrate or make decisions and can cause you to feel disconnected from your baby and to isolate from others. It can also cause intense worry and anxiety about your infant's health or your ability to care for your baby.

Fearing you're unable to care for your baby is much different than having thoughts, hallucinations, or delusions about harming your baby. These severe symptoms are a medical emergency and should be treated as such. If you are having scary thoughts of any kind, please reach out to your medical provider or consult the Resources section (page 146).

Finding your way through this time can be difficult, but it is temporary and with help you will feel better. You are already taking action. It's crucial to take small steps that build new habits and support, such as those included in this journal. As a new parent, work on cultivating greater compassion for yourself, finding comfort and understanding, and accepting that there is no such thing as a perfect parent. This section will help you learn to cope with challenging emotions while gaining confidence in your parenting.

IDENTIFYING
EMOTIONS

And one has to understand that braveness is not the absence of fear but rather the strength to keep on going forward despite the fear.

—Paulo Coelho

YOUR EMOTIONS

There are five core emotions: joy, fear, sadness, disgust, and anger. Notice that only one is commonly regarded as positive; the rest are usually labeled negative. People often discuss the joy that pregnancy and parenting bring. Most new parents are frightened when negative emotions prevail or positive ones are missing altogether. How do you respond when a negative emotion pops up? Is it easier or harder to accept than positive emotions? What could the negative emotion be trying to signal to you?

EXAMINING YOUR EMOTIONS

You can feel any core emotion with differing levels of intensity. The intensity itself can create a new emotion and expand into hundreds of nuances. For example, sadness may include agony, hurt, helplessness, and fragility. Share the prevalent emotions you've experienced over the past 24 hours. Did any of them grow, change, or react to other feelings?

Legs Up the Wall

There are many practices that facilitate relaxation and benefit both your mind and body by slowing breathing rate, relaxing muscles, and reducing blood pressure. Legs up the wall is a relatively simple yoga pose that looks just like its name. If you have glaucoma, a hernia, a heart condition, or limited mobility, or if the posture isn't comfortable, feel free to choose a different movement. Simple stretching and slowing your breathing can help you relax.

1. Place a yoga mat or blanket on the floor next to a wall, with a small pillow for your head if needed.

2. Lie down on the mat with your tailbone flat on the floor, a few inches from the wall, and stretch your legs up against the wall.

3. The backs of your legs should be flush with the wall. Flex your feet so they're parallel to the floor. Relax your knees. You should feel a light stretch, but it shouldn't be painful.

4. Relax and breathe deeply. Try and stay in the pose for two or three minutes, or as long as you're comfortable.

5. To exit the pose, move carefully into a comfortable seated position, and sit quietly for at least 30 seconds before standing.

What did you notice after trying this yoga pose? Any changes in your heart rate, or overall relaxation?

CORE EMOTIONS

Noticing and naming your emotions makes it easier to accept and live with them. Using the chart of emotions on page 58, notice where the emotions you identified on page 55 are located. Do they cluster around one core emotion, or are they evenly dispersed? Notice how two emotions like anger and disgust meet and create contempt. Make an expanded list of your emotions.

1. _____

2. _____

3. _____

4. _____

5. _____

6. _____

7. _____

8. _____

9. _____

10. _____

11. _____

12. _____

13. _____

14. _____

15. _____

	JOY	FEAR	SADNESS	DISGUST	ANGER
HIGH INTENSITY	Blissful Ecstatic Grateful Inspired Surprised	Surprised Frightened Threatened Remorseful	Remorseful Angry Distressed Agonized Ashamed	Ashamed Abused Contemptuous	Contemptuous Furious Enraged Hateful Outraged
	Happy Passionate Fulfilled Awed Enthusiastic Satisfied Hopeful Excited Proud Admiring Courageous	Scared Nervous Shocked Vigilant Afraid Unsafe Intimidated Angry Dreading Desperate	Anxious Regretful Rejected Heartbroken Depressed Helpless Worthless Lonely	Nauseated Humiliated Guilty Jealous Alienated Betrayed	Bitter Aggressive Livid Frantic Violated Frustrated
LOW INTENSITY	Brave Powerful Energetic Creative Confident Curious Cheerful Affectionate Eager Caring Determined	Concerned Distrustful Paranoid Overwhelmed Humble Stunned Timid Challenged Defensive Conflicted Indecisive	Empty Abandoned Fragile Disappointed Pessimistic Shy Crushed Hopeless Isolated Inconsolable	Embarrassed Envious Discouraged Ignored Awkward Disturbed Incompetent Coerced Deprived Apathetic Diminished	Mad Irritated Resentful Aggravated Vindictive Offended Insulted Spiteful Provoked Antagonized

FEELING YOUR EMOTIONS

Think about your most recent experience with joy, or any of the related emotions you identified. What thoughts come to mind? Where do you experience joy in your body as you think about these memories? Do you welcome the sensation or try to suppress it?

FEELING ALL YOUR EMOTIONS

Identify one of the more challenging emotions you've been struggling with. See if you can notice where you experience this emotion in your body. Do you welcome the sensation or try to suppress it? How long can you sit with this feeling?

FIGHT, FLIGHT, OR FREEZE

Fight, flight, or freeze is your body's natural response to a perceived threat. Many present-day moments can trigger the response and subsequently release stress hormones. Think back to a recent time when you felt stressed or overwhelmed. What sensations did you experience in your body? What specific circumstances made you feel threatened or unsafe?

RELAXATION RESPONSE

The opposite of the fight-flight-or-freeze response is the relaxation response, which allows your mind and body to rebalance, reduce stress, and find a sense of peace. What activities, including practices in this book, help you feel calm and relaxed? What sensations do you notice in your body when you are relaxed? How can you incorporate relaxation techniques when you are feeling a flight-fight-or-freeze reaction?

Accepting Difficult Emotions Through Mindfulness

It's common to avoid uncomfortable emotions. Some people use alcohol or drugs to numb their feelings. Others exercise, overeat, or choose not to eat. Crying, yelling, avoiding others, and being self-critical are all ways of coping with difficult emotions, thoughts, or memories. Developing a mindfulness practice can teach you how to acknowledge your thoughts, feelings, and memories without letting them derail you. Mindfulness is the practice of noticing that your attention has wandered to a thought or feeling and redirecting it to wherever you want it to be, like your breath, an object, or a mantra. Mindfulness also means you don't judge yourself for any thoughts or feelings. Start by picking a mundane task like changing your baby's diaper or taking a shower. If you notice your mind wander, bring your attention back to the task at hand—taking a wipe out of the box or feeling hot water hit your face. You may find your mind wanders a lot. It is normal. Your job is to bring your attention back—without judging yourself.

MINDFULNESS AND YOU

What mundane task did you focus on for the mindfulness practice? Was it easy to maintain focus? What thoughts came up? Were there any feelings? Memories? Was it difficult to bring your attention back to the activity you were doing? Remember mindfulness doesn't solve your problems, but it helps you learn to cope with difficult feelings, thoughts, and memories.

BENEFITS OF MINDFULNESS

Mindfulness teaches you to notice your thoughts, feelings, and emotions, then acknowledge them and let them go as you return to the present moment. Practicing mindfulness regularly helps you pause before responding and teaches you that emotions come and go, like waves in the ocean rising and falling. Have you noticed your own emotions ebb and flow in this way? What would it be like if you could pause before you react?

MINDFULNESS IN EVERYDAY LIFE

As a new parent, it's difficult to imagine making time to do one more thing. Mindfulness can be part of your everyday life and doesn't require silence or special equipment. What's most important to remember is that mindfulness is a practice, and the greatest benefits will come from making it part of your daily routine. Make a list of the mundane tasks you can practice doing mindfully.

1. _____

2. _____

3. _____

4. _____

5. _____

6. _____

7. _____

8. _____

9. _____

10. _____

11. _____

12. _____

13. _____

14. _____

15. _____

RAIN

RAIN is a structured mindfulness and self-compassion practice. This version, modified by psychologist Tara Brach, is incredibly effective for working with intense or difficult emotions. I recommend a guided meditation if this practice is new for you. Please see the Resources section (page 146) to find a recording. RAIN is an acronym for the four steps of the process:

(R) Recognize what is happening. What's going on inside you? What are your physical sensations, emotions, thoughts, and feelings? Identify what is happening in the present moment, such as, *"I'm feeling like a failure after my baby screamed all morning and I couldn't calm them down."*

(A) Allow things to be just as they are. Allowing the thoughts, emotions, feelings, or sensations you recognized to just be there doesn't mean you have to like the situation.

(I) Investigate the emotions you've recognized. Become curious about them and how they feel in your body. Notice how the feelings are affecting you.

(N) Nurture yourself; see if you can offer yourself what you need. Perhaps it is gentle words of comfort, or something you need from someone else. Can you imagine someone fulfilling that need for you?

After practicing RAIN, notice any shifts within. Do you feel lighter, calmer, and more relaxed in your body?

IDENTITY

Between stimulus and response there is a space. In that space is our power to choose our response. In our response lies our growth and our freedom.

—Viktor E. Frankl

Butterfly Hug

The butterfly hug, which comes from eye movement desensitization and reprocessing (EMDR) therapy, will help you feel grounded, lower your heart rate, and decrease anxiety.

1. Make yourself comfortable. Stand up, sit in a chair, or lie down, eyes open or closed.

2. Start by crossing your hands across your chest, hooking your thumbs, and allowing your middle fingers (the butterfly wings) to rest just below your collarbone.

3. Slowly tap your left hand on your chest, then your right hand, alternating sides until you find a rhythm that feels good.

4. Breathe in and out through your nose until you start to feel calmer.

5. Notice whether your body feels calmer.

The butterfly hug is great because you can do it anywhere and you'll notice the effects in less than a minute, although I recommend taking at least a few moments to enjoy the calming effects. It is a great tool when you have physical sensations of anxiety like a racing heart, insomnia, sweating, or shortness of breath, or you're feeling jittery, like you've had too much caffeine.

How did you feel about the butterfly hug? Did you sense the calming effects in your body? How likely are you to try it again?

_____

_____

_____

_____

_____

_____

YOUR PARENTING EXPECTATIONS

What messages did you receive from society, the media, and your family about how parenthood would and should look? What has been harder or easier than you'd imagined? What do you wish you had known before you became a parent?

MYTHS OF PARENTHOOD

Society and media send messages that parenting will come naturally: the baby will easily suckle at the breast and sleep peacefully when laid down, and parents will intuitively know what their baby needs by the sound of their cry. These messages become expectations, but they are truly myths. List five myths of parenthood you wish you had known weren't true before your baby arrived.

THE FANTASY

The mundane tasks of parenthood can challenge one's idealized view of parenting. The image of a baby sleeping peacefully rarely translates to the real world. More often, tired parents are forced to reconcile what it means to be completely obsessed with sleep. For others, the issue is not sleep but feeding, or soothing a fussy baby. How have you experienced the divergence between the fantasy and the reality of parenting?

SHIFTING IDENTITY

Before your baby arrived, you likely slept when you were tired, ate when you were hungry, and used the bathroom when needed—and now all that looks very different. What is it like to have your world upended and to lose that independence? What parts of your old life do you miss?

WHO WERE YOU?

Who were you before you became a parent? Did you work? Were you a student? What did you do with your free time? How did you introduce yourself at a party? How have you introduced yourself since your baby was born? How has your identity shifted since becoming a parent?

YOUR EMOTIONS AND YOUR IDENTITY SHIFT

For new parents, the freedom and independence that once defined you suddenly evaporate. What emotions come up as you think about the loss of the old you and your old life? Notice where you feel the emotions in your body. What are these emotions trying to tell you?

SHAME

Shame is the feeling of being flawed and therefore unworthy of love and belonging, according to researcher Brené Brown. New parents may experience shame for many reasons, including missing your old life; having negative feelings about your baby; feeling consumed by sadness, anxiety, or fear; or desperately wanting a baby and finding it less fulfilling than imagined. Sometimes it's a mix of all these reasons and more. Share your experience with shame.

If you put shame in a petri dish, it needs three things to grow exponentially: secrecy, silence and judgment. If you put the same amount in a petri dish and douse it with empathy, it can't survive. The two most powerful words when we're in struggle: me too.

—Brené Brown

Thoughts, Behavior, and Emotions

Cognitive behavioral therapy (CBT) is based on the understanding that what you think influences how you feel, and your thinking isn't always accurate. CBT teaches you how to examine your thoughts and work with them in ways that improve mood and encourage you to be realistic.

For example, a new friend invited Sara to join a group of other parents at the park over the weekend. Sara declined (behavior), fearful that they wouldn't like her (thoughts) or that her baby was difficult because he cried so much. She was sad and lonely on Saturday (feelings).

Imagine what might have happened if Sara told herself instead, "Maybe I'll meet some new friends and have a good time" or "Maybe someone else is also struggling with a fussy baby and it's not just me." If she had gone to the park, how could things have been different? She likely wouldn't have felt lonely and perhaps she would have felt more connected to others.

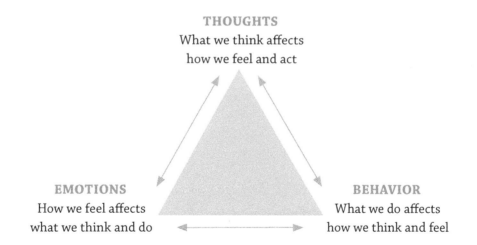

THOUGHTS
What we think affects
how we feel and act

EMOTIONS
How we feel affects
what we think and do

BEHAVIOR
What we do affects
how we think and feel

Reflect on a recent time when you were feeling sad or anxious. Recall your thoughts at that time.

How did you feel about the situation?

What was your behavior? How did your thoughts or feelings impact your behavior?

How would this situation have been different if you had been aware of the impact of your thoughts?

Try paying attention to your thoughts for the next few days and then come back and share what you learned.

ISOLATION AND LONELINESS

Feelings of sadness, anxiety, fear, and shame often make it harder to care for a baby, not to mention carry out everyday tasks. As a result, many new parents find themselves increasingly isolated and lonely, which tends to fuel symptoms and create distance from their old self. Share how your postpartum depression has impacted your relationships and interactions with others.

There is no agony like bearing an untold story inside you.

—Zora Neale Hurston

Expressive Journaling

Research shows a positive connection between expressive journal writing and improved mental and physical health. Although scientists can't say exactly why writing about your emotions is valuable, the consensus is that telling stories helps, and it's beneficial to use the words *understand*, *realize*, and *because*. Get a blank journal or notebook and try these six steps to get started:

1. **Carve out time.** You don't have to journal every day, but aim for 15 minutes three to four days a week.

2. **Experiment with your method.** Handwrite or use a phone or a computer. You can even record yourself speaking.

3. **Find the right place.** Where you write can affect your feelings. The most important thing is to have a quiet place.

4. **Don't edit yourself.** Access your feelings and allow yourself to flow. Leave out the punctuation; make mistakes! The goal is self-expression, not perfection.

5. **Write about any experience that is important to you.**

6. **Reread.** Your writing is a record of your life. Go back and see what you've written. You may want to rewrite it or you may want to rip it up. Your choice!

What was it like to write your thoughts and feelings on paper rather than keeping them in your head? Is it different than sharing them with someone verbally?

HEALING

REFLECTING ON YOUR EXPECTATIONS

Look back at Your Parenting Expectations (page 71) and notice the expectations you had for yourself as a parent. What would you say to your best friend, sibling, or child about the transition to parenthood? Share what you would tell them if they held those same expectations.

A GOOD ENOUGH PARENT

What if you told yourself *"I'm a good enough parent"*? For a moment, ask the part of you that wants to challenge that statement to step aside. Now repeat the phrase *"I'm a good enough parent."* Share what it feels like to believe for just a moment that your love and effort is more than enough and your baby is lucky to have you.

REFLECTING ON PRIOR TRANSITIONS

Remember a time you started a new job or school. Recall finding your classes, turning in your first assignment, or making your first presentation. Notice your emotions. What helped you feel confident and secure? Share how that experience reminds you of what you're experiencing as a new parent. What kindness can you show yourself now as you navigate this transition?

ATTUNING TO YOUR SUCCESS

Just as your earlier adjustment to a new school or job required time before you felt comfortable, your newborn was a stranger at first. You didn't know how your baby liked to be fed or cuddled. Celebrate three things you have learned about your baby and celebrate your growth as a parent.

I'm not afraid of storms, for I am learning how to sail my ship.

—Louisa May Alcott

Values Exercise

The life compass is an exercise used in acceptance and commitment therapy (ACT). It can clarify values by helping you explore specific qualities. This exercise can help you tease out exactly what *good* means. What qualities define this word for you? Compassionate? Trustworthy? Fun? You can use this exercise to explore the words provided or any of your own.

1. Write a few words about what is important or meaningful to you about parenting. What kind of parent do you want to be? What qualities or strengths do you want to cultivate and model with your baby? How do you want to behave? Review the list for ideas, but choose the words that mean the most to you.

2. In the upper right corner of the box, on a scale of 0 to 10 mark how important your chosen values are at this point in your life if 0 = no importance and 10 = extremely important.

3. In the lower right corner, on a scale of 0 to 10 mark how effectively you're living by these values right now if 0 = not at all and 10 = living by them fully.

Accepting	Fun	Self-caring
Adventurous	Generous	Trusting
Assertive	Grateful	Trustworthy
Authentic	Honest	Other _____
Caring	Loving	_____
Compassionate	Mindful	
Creative	Reliable	
Empathic	Respectful	
Forgiving	Responsible	

PARENTING

WORK

RELATIONSHIPS

OTHER

YOUR VALUES AS A PARENT

What did you learn about your values as a parent from this exercise?

_____

_____

_____

_____

_____

_____

_____

_____

_____

_____

_____

_____

_____

_____

_____

_____

_____

_____

_____

CLARIFYING YOUR VALUES

Identifying values can help you move in the direction you want to go and get in the practice of living those values in your daily life. If the values exercise was difficult, try answering these questions: What do the fears, worries, and anxieties you identified in Core Emotions (page 57) show that you care about? What do they remind you is important?

LIVING IN ALIGNMENT WITH YOUR VALUES

Reflecting on the values you've identified previously, what is one thing you can do to live in greater alignment to those values?

4-7-8 Breathing

The 4-7-8 breathing technique helps decrease stress, calm anxiety, and improve sleep. It forces you to focus solely on your breath, taking your attention away from stressful thoughts while calming your mind and relaxing your body.

You can do this exercise anywhere at any time, although it's recommended to sit with a straight back to allow your lungs enough space to expand.

1. Start by taking a few deep breaths. Then exhale completely, emptying the lungs of air.

2. If comfortable, close your eyes.

3. Breathe in through your nose as you count to four. Be sure to let your belly expand as you inhale.

4. Pause your breath for a count of seven.

5. Exhale through your mouth to the count of eight.

6. Repeat for four full cycles.

7. Practice this breathing technique two times per day.

This exercise can calm and relax you quickly, but the effects are also cumulative. After about six weeks, you'll start to notice more significant positive effects, like better sleep and lowered blood pressure.

New breathing techniques may cause you to feel slightly light-headed. If it happens, take a break until you're comfortable starting again.

Reflect on your experience with 4-7-8 breathing. Will you commit to trying this practice to reap the long-term benefits? If not, why not?

PART 3

Changing Relationships, Expectations, and Self-Identity

Feeling anxious or depressed about the birth of a child is a huge shock for most new parents. You may feel shame and fear for struggling during a time you think you should feel joyful.

Know that you are not alone. Becoming a parent is likely the biggest adjustment you have experienced as an adult. Recognizing feelings of shame and fear and developing strategies to process them can help you understand yourself and develop the capacity to heal your pain and become the parent you were meant to be.

RELATIONSHIPS

All changes, even the most longed for, have their melancholy; for what we leave behind us is a part of ourselves; we must die to one life before we can enter another.

—Anatole France

YOUR PRE-BABY RELATIONSHIP WITH YOUR PARTNER

What was your relationship with your partner like before your baby arrived? How did you spend your time together? What were your interactions like? Did you fight much? How did you resolve conflict? What was the chemistry like between you two?

NEW RELATIONSHIP CHALLENGES

Many couples assume a baby will bring them closer or improve their relationship. Research shows, however, that two-thirds of couples report a decrease in marital satisfaction during the first three years of parenthood. How did you imagine your relationship would change, if at all? Has your relationship evolved as you predicted?

FEELING TOUCHED OUT

As a parent of an infant, you're their lifeline, and they need attention throughout the day and night. Those who are breastfeeding or chestfeeding share their body with their baby, further depleting themselves physically. What is the emotional toll of caregiving for you? Do you ever feel overwhelmed by physical contact? What does being "touched out" feel like, and how does it impact your relationship with your partner?

Protecting Your Relationship

Although your children are an important part of your family, they're not the only important part. Children need to grow up seeing that all members of their family are valued, respected, and appreciated. How you treat and feel about each other as parents models what a relationship is for your children.

Assess your relationship, sharing your reflections for each topic. Consider sharing these prompts with your partner and discussing your responses together.

Communication: You talk about stuff—not just which stroller or diaper you need, but the deeper stuff. You discuss issues such as what you liked and disliked about your own childhood and want to replicate and avoid and how the adjustment is going.

Intimacy: You feel connected to each other. How have you maintained your physical connection? Did you discuss how birth might impact your sex life and have you touched base about how to stay connected until you're both ready?

Respect: You feel your opinions are heard and equally valued. Caring for a new baby can bring out passionate viewpoints that we didn't anticipate. It's important to remain open to our partner's ideas and values.

_____

_____

_____

Caretaking: You take care of each other. Waking up a million times a night means someone may need a nap. Do you look out for each other?

_____

_____

_____

THE MENTAL LOAD OF PARENTING

It's only in recent times that parenting has become more of a shared responsibility. Being the primary parent who carries the mental load of child-rearing can be taxing, however, especially when you're struggling with depression or anxiety. Make a list of five things your partner can do every day to help out.

1. _____

_____

2. _____

_____

3. _____

_____

4. _____

_____

5. _____

_____

ASKING FOR HELP

It can be difficult to ask for help when you're feeling down. Enlisting support from your community can be life-changing, whether it's cooking or cleaning from friends or family, help finding a therapist, or hiring someone to cover the night shift so you can sleep. Where do you need support right now? Who can you ask for help, or to help you get the support you need?

Joy shared twice the gain, sorrow shared half the pain.

—Swedish proverb

RELATIONSHIP WITH FAMILY

What was your relationship like with your parents and in-laws before your baby arrived? What kinds of boundaries and expectations existed? Did they drop in unannounced? Did they respect your privacy? Share the kind of support you were hoping for when you announced you were expecting a baby versus how things are going now.

_____

_____

_____

_____

_____

_____

_____

_____

_____

_____

_____

_____

_____

_____

_____

_____

_____

FAMILY SUPPORT

Having family that live around the corner can be both helpful and challenging for new parents. Likewise, having family across the country comes with its own pluses and minuses. How has your family supported you through this transition? How can they be more helpful? Do you need more space, someone to fold the laundry, someone to hold the baby, someone to listen?

PARENTING CHOICES

Some new parents have clear ideas about how they will raise their child. How would you like to parent your child? How have your ideas changed? Is there an internal pressure to repeat or reject the way you were parented?

_____

_____

_____

_____

_____

_____

_____

_____

_____

_____

_____

_____

_____

_____

_____

_____

MAINTAINING FRIENDSHIPS

Maintaining friendships as you transition to parenthood can require an enormous effort. The shift from your old life and distance from friends can feel isolating, which exacerbates stress and sadness. Have you managed to maintain connection with your old friends? How can you increase your social connections?

Relationship Map

A relationship map allows you to visually explore your support system. Use the circle diagram, along with the following prompts, to help you complete your map.

1. Write your own name in the middle of the smallest circle.

2. Identify 8 to 10 people in your life who are most important. Write their names, placing those who are closest to you toward the center.

3. Reflect on what it felt like to create this map, and how it feels as you look at it.

4. Circle the names of the people who bring the most positivity into your life.

5. Underline those who create issues for you, drain your energy, or deplete your spirits.

6. Would you like to make any changes in your relationship life?

7. Who is not in the circle that you wish was?

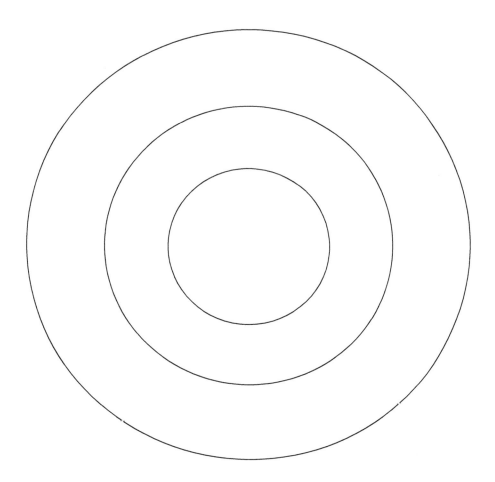

EXPECTATIONS AND PRESSURES IN PARENTING

To be beautiful means to be yourself. You don't need to be accepted by others. You need to accept yourself.

—Thich Nhat Hanh

EMBRACING THE BODY YOU HAVE

It takes about a year for a postpartum body to return to its prepregnancy shape. Comparing yourself to others often contributes to negative feelings about your own self-worth. Take a moment and look into your eyes in a mirror. Find something about your body you can cherish and feel grateful for and write about it.

SOCIAL MEDIA: BEWARE THE URGE TO COMPARE

It's human nature to compare yourself to others. Unfortunately, social media posts of smiling parents with spotless homes and choreographed photo shoots from the pumpkin patch can make you feel like you or your life is inadequate. Make a list of social media accounts and contacts that leave you feeling down or depressed. Which can you unfollow or mute?

AN INSTAGRAM BLESSING: #SPEAKTHESECRET

Social media can also be helpful. Which accounts do you follow that make you laugh, smile, and feel seen? Check out #SpeakTheSecret on Instagram and see what it's like to join a community who shares your struggle. Share three things that you find memorable or inspirational about this hashtag.

Reclaim Joyful, Positive Experiences

Even if you're having a stressful time right now, you have undoubtedly had times in your life that were not filled with the pain and anxiety of postpartum depression. Being able to access positive experiences and moments of joy will help you heal.

1. Find a quiet place where you can breathe deeply and reflect.

2. Recall an activity that you once enjoyed or a time you had fun. Can you find a moment you were smiling or laughing with a friend? Perhaps you enjoyed hiking in the woods or reading a good book. Perhaps you had fun going shopping and out for lunch. Maybe dancing, knitting, or cooking was your thing.

3. See yourself having positive experiences and notice what that feels like in your body. Is there anyone you might call to reminisce about these fun times?

4. Fast forward and imagine you're able to participate in one of these activities again.

5. Write about what has come up for you as you reclaim positive experiences to help you get through the challenges of today.

UNREALISTIC EXPECTATIONS

Taking care of a new baby is a full-time job that's physically, mentally, and emotionally taxing. Society, however, may lead you to believe that caring for children is a simple, easy, stress-free, and relaxing activity. How does this misperception make you feel? Do you find yourself getting angry when people underestimate how much work parenting is?

_____

_____

_____

_____

_____

_____

_____

_____

_____

_____

_____

_____

_____

_____

_____

_____

MANAGING YOUR WORKLOAD

Some new parents work outside the home. Others stay home or work part time and use the remaining time for childcare. How did you decide what you would do? Was it always the plan or did plans change after your baby arrived? How do you feel about your responsibilities working inside or outside the home, or doing both?

FEELINGS ABOUT WORK

Some new parents experience grief or guilt with separation from their child, whereas others are invigorated by the change of schedule and the break of being apart. What has your experience been? What feelings arise as you think about it?

*And, now that you don't have to be perfect,
you can be good.*

—John Steinbeck

BONDING WITH YOUR BABY

Although most new parents anticipate feeling bonded to their baby from birth, up to 20 percent feel no immediate connection to their baby for hours, weeks, or months. PMADs can interfere with bonding, often leaving new parents disappointed, confused, or ashamed. Share about your connection with your baby.

Bonding Through Massage

Infant massage can benefit those struggling with postpartum depression, facilitating relaxation and bonding through eye contact, smiling, soothing noises, gentle touch, and interaction.

1. Find a comfortable spot in a warm room (~75°F). Use the time to talk or sing to your baby.

2. Follow your baby's cues. If your baby appears calm and content, they might enjoy a massage. If they turn their head away or become stiff in your arms, consider waiting.

3. Slowly stroke and knead each part of your baby's body.

4. Place your baby on their back and begin by rubbing each body part, starting with their head and moving down to their feet.

5. No specific amount of time is recommended; the massage should last as long as you and your baby are enjoying it. You can try placing your baby on their belly, although some may not tolerate this position for long.

6. Watch how your baby responds. If your baby seems happy, continue. If they turn their head away or appear restless or unhappy, stop and try later.

7. Reflect on your experience connecting with your baby through massage.

STRENGTHENING THE PARENT-BABY BOND

There are many ways to increase bonding. Some examples include:

- Massage
- Looking in their eyes while feeding
- Kangaroo care or holding your baby skin-to-skin
- Reading or singing to baby
- Carrying your baby in your arms or in a baby carrier
- Mimicking your baby's sounds

Using this list and your own research, reflect on ways you are already bonding with your baby and come up with ideas for strengthening your connection.

_____

_____

_____

_____

_____

_____

_____

_____

_____

_____

_____

Shame and PMADs

Shame is the feeling of being flawed and unworthy of love and belonging. Often people experiencing postpartum depression or anxiety stay silent because of the shame of struggling during a time they feel should be joyful. They find themselves feeling trapped, powerless, or isolated, which further exacerbates symptoms of postpartum depression. Empathy, connection, power, and freedom are the well-proven anecdotes to shame. Shame needs to be acknowledged and understood before it can be overcome. Shame resilience theory (SRT) suggests that shame is most harmful when it goes unacknowledged. Watch Brené Brown's YouTube video "The Power of Vulnerability." Come back and reflect on your own experience with shame. What are your initial reactions to the video?

DEVELOPING
RESILIENCE

In giving birth to our babies, we may find that we give birth to new possibilities within ourselves.

—Myla and Jon Kabat-Zinn

BUILDING SHAME RESILIENCE

Shame resilience theory teaches you to respond to shame by recognizing your internal and external triggers and discussing your feelings with others. Shame is universal, and it shows up when you feel that you fail to measure up to others' expectations. Take a moment to recall a time you experienced and shared something shameful with a friend, relative, or neighbor. What was your experience sharing?

_____

_____

_____

_____

_____

_____

_____

_____

_____

_____

_____

_____

_____

_____

_____

_____

SHARING WITH SOMEONE YOU TRUST

It's important to identify a person who is likely to be supportive and empathic. Scan your world of friends, colleagues, family, and neighbors. Can you identify anyone who has offered you support in the past? Imagine taking a risk and sharing what you're going through. Write about what you hope will happen.

UNDERSTANDING VULNERABILITY

Researcher Brené Brown defines vulnerability as "uncertainty, risk, and emotional exposure." It's that shaky feeling that comes up when you think about doing something out of your comfort zone. Vulnerability is often misunderstood as weakness, but it's actually the opposite: It takes courage to show up and be seen. Share what it would look like to be more vulnerable.

Practicing Vulnerability

Whether it's sharing your feelings with your partner, attending a new parent support group, or telling someone you've been struggling, courage is required. And the payoff is worth it: developing deeper connections, feeling less isolated, and being your true authentic self. But how do you get started?

Notice the feeling of vulnerability in your body. Acknowledge and truly experience any uncomfortable sensations. Do not try to avoid or numb them. Getting used to them will make it easier to sit in vulnerability.

Push yourself outside your comfort zone. What would that be for you? Joining a music class with your baby? Asking a parent at the park to join you for coffee? Maybe it's telling your mother-in-law you need help.

Share your truth. This practice is the foundational essence of vulnerability. Share your accomplishments, your fears, your love, your feelings of shame and insecurity. Share it all with people you trust.

Practice. Becoming more vulnerable takes practice. You have to notice your discomfort and put yourself out there anyway. Eventually the fear of rejection or judgment will seem insignificant and following your own heart will become more natural.

You don't ever have to do anything sensational for people to love you.

—Fred Rogers

PRACTICING GRATITUDE

Gratitude can help protect against dark thoughts and negative attitudes and improve physical health and sleep. Focus on something small that has been positive for you recently, like washing your hair or brushing your teeth. Notice what it feels like in your body and share your reflections.

DEVELOPING SELF-COMPASSION

Imagine seeing a friend sitting in a rainstorm and handing them an umbrella. Now imagine seeing yourself instead of the friend and handing yourself the same umbrella. That sensation is what self-compassion looks like. Notice what you are feeling in your body. Write about what it is like to be both the receiver and the giver.

UNDERSTANDING GUILT AND SHAME

Shame and guilt are often confused. Guilt, the feeling that you *did* something bad, can be a productive emotion that motivates you to repair your mistakes. Shame, on the other hand, is the feeling that you *are* bad. Shame is more challenging to address, and it often stems from long-held negative beliefs. How have guilt and shame come up since you became a parent?

Self-Compassion and Shame

Shame is rooted in negative core beliefs ("I'm bad, unworthy, unlovable") that cannot be easily repaired like guilt. Shame causes you to dismiss your value and question your worth. Self-compassion allows you to experience your feelings without getting trapped by shame.

Can you remember a recent time when you felt shame? What was it like? Did you want to withdraw, blame someone, or lash out? As you reflect on that experience, try this self-compassion practice:

- **Mindfulness:** Acknowledge your feelings or thoughts of shame. Pay attention to where the sensations of shame show up in your body or acknowledge your thoughts about being inadequate, defective, or unworthy. Now name the experience the way you would for a friend.
- **Common humanity:** Remind yourself that everyone experiences shame. It is human to feel shame and you're not alone.
- **Self-kindness:** Approach your experience with tenderness. Remind yourself that shame emerges from your universal human need to be loved.

Reflect on your experience. Remind yourself you're still a good person despite feelings of inadequacy. You don't need to be perfect to fit in or be loved. Notice any shifts in how you feel. This self-compassion practice can be helpful in coping with any number of distressing thoughts and behaviors, whether you're feeling shame, irritability, or sadness.

NOTICING WHAT WORKS

Keeping a journal can bring new thoughts and feelings to the surface. You may discover you're worried about something you weren't aware of until you wrote it down. You may notice new patterns. You may find writing helps you feel more in charge of your life. What have you learned through this journal so far?

INCREASING SUPPORT

Scan over the prompts on pages 109–113 about relationships. How varied is your support network? Do you know other new parents with babies of similar age? Do you know anyone overcoming a PMAD? Search Postpartum Support International to find a local in-person or virtual support group. What would it be like to receive support from others who get it?

STRUGGLES ARE OPPORTUNITIES

Struggles offer you the opportunity to recognize your strengths and resources and to build new ones. Hopefully you have had a chance to create or strengthen your internal and external toolbox of resources through using this journal. Jot down three strategies you have found useful. What did you like about them? How can you incorporate them into your life?

RADICAL ACCEPTANCE

Pretending everything is okay takes a lot of work and can be utterly exhausting. Radical acceptance is about recognizing the present moment without judgment. With acknowledgment and acceptance, pain often dissipates. Speaking your feelings aloud validates your experiences, and when you face your emotions their intensity softens. What feelings have you been ignoring or suppressing? How can you start accepting them instead?

Plan

Accepting a diagnosis of a PMAD can be difficult and requires a shift in expectations and perception. You may not have been prepared, but you must adapt to allow yourself to move forward. You have a new baby to care for and you must take care of yourself as well. You must hold a number of concepts that you may not have been concerned with in the past. It's important to bring self-compassion to the forefront. Self-compassion is an internal process, so you may need to remind yourself that you didn't do anything wrong to cause this situation, but you will feel better if you deal with it. Accepting your feelings and determining what you can control will help. Creating and sticking to an action plan to eat nourishing food, get more sleep, find ways to move your body that feel good, and socialize—in person or virtually—are key. Write down specific ways you can ensure self-care remains a part of your routine. What are three things you'd like to continue or start doing each day? Each week? Which friends or family members can you enlist to help you make time and stick to your plan?

1. _____

_____

2. _____

_____

3. _____

_____

FINAL NOTE

You've put in a great deal of effort toward healing your postpartum depression. Having the courage to use this journal is an important step in recovery. My hope is that you have started to feel better physically, emotionally, and mentally.

Building and maintaining your support system is crucial to navigating this difficult season. Yes, this is a season, and it will pass. I hope you have begun to envision your life without postpartum depression. With support and commitment, as you've shown here, you *will* feel better.

It is normal to experience setbacks. They are an inevitable part of the journey, not a sign of failure. Returning to work and weaning from breastfeeding or chestfeeding are common times when postpartum depression may resurface. Leaning on others and using the new strategies you have practiced can help you manage difficult physical and emotional symptoms when they occur. Note which journal exercises have been particularly useful and return to them when you need to.

Acknowledge your vulnerability, strength, and courage, which have been called on to address this challenging, unanticipated, and unwelcomed season in your life. Recognize your resilience and what a wonderful model you are for your child: a dedicated parent who prioritizes their own health and wellness.

Please consult the resource section of this journal for books, websites, apps, and online communities that can offer you additional support today and throughout your parenting journey. Congratulations on your hard work!

RESOURCES

Information and Support

Postpartum Support International offers a provider directory to connect with perinatal therapists, virtually or in person. It hosts free virtual support groups for parents. PostPartum.net

EMDRIA is a professional association for practitioners trained in eye movement desensitization and reprocessing (EMDR), an evidence-based trauma therapy. EMDRIA hosts a provider directory. Emdria.org

Somatic Experiencing is an organization that trains mind–body therapists in treating trauma. TraumaHealing.org

Postpartum Progress offers blogs, articles, and resources. PostpartumProgress.com

Mindfulness Audio Recordings

UCSD Center for Mindfulness
CIH.UCSD.edu/mindfulness

UCLA Mindful Awareness Research Center
UCLAHealth.org/marc

Kristin Neff, a pioneer in self-compassion research and practices
Self-Compassion.org

Mindfulness Apps

New Gratitude Journal

Calm

Insight Timer

Mind the Bump

Expectful

Mindful IVF

Books

Down Came the Rain: My Journey Through Postpartum Depression, by Brooke Shields

Emotional Agility: Get Unstuck, Embrace Change, and Thrive in Work and Life, by Susan David

The Gifts of Imperfect Parenting: Raising Children with Courage, Compassion, and Connection, by Brené Brown

Good Moms Have Scary Thoughts: A Healing Guide to the Secret Fears of New Mothers, by Karen Kleiman

The Happiness Trap: How to Stop Struggling and Start Living: A Guide to ACT, by Russ Harris

The Joy of Parenting: An Acceptance and Commitment Therapy Guide to Effective Parenting in the Early Years, by Lisa Coyne and Amy R. Murrell

This Isn't What I Expected: Overcoming Postpartum Depression, by Karen Kleiman

What About Us? A New Parent's Guide to Safeguarding Your Over-Anxious, Over-Extended, Sleep-Deprived Relationship, by Karen Kleiman and Molly McIntyre

Women's Moods: What Every Woman Must Know About Hormones, the Brain, and Emotional Health, by Deborah Sichel and Jeanne Watson Driscoll

Instagram

@blackmamasmatter
@drcassidy
@drsterlingobgyn
@momandmind (and her podcast by the same name)
@mother.ly
@postpartumstress
@shadesofblueproject

REFERENCES

Alcott, Louisa May. *Little Women*. New York: Penguin Books, 2021.

Brown, Brené. *Daring Greatly: How the Courage to Be Vulnerable Transforms the Way We Live, Love, Parent, and Lead*. New York: Avery Publishing Group, 2015.

Brown, Brené. "*Listening to Shame*." (2012) TED.com/talks/brene_brown_listening _to_shame (accessed June 6, 2021).

Coelho, Paulo. PauloCoelhoBlog.com/2011/08/25/doubt-and-fear-editar (accessed December 8, 2021).

Gottman, Jon and Julie Schwartz Gottman. *And Baby Makes Three: The Six-Step Plan for Preserving Marital Intimacy and Rekindling Romance After Baby Arrives*. New York: Three Rivers Press, 2008.

Harris, Russ. *ACT Made Simple: An Easy-to-Read Primer on Acceptance and Commitment Therapy*. Oakland, CA: New Harbinger Publications, Inc., 2019.

Hurston, Zora Neale. *Dust Tracks on a Road: Autobiography*. London: Virago Press, 1986.

Keller, Helen. *Optimism*. Boston: D. B. Updike, The Merrymount Press, 1903.

Kleiman, Karen. *Good Moms Have Scary Thoughts: A Healing Guide to the Secret Fears of New Mothers*. New York: Familius, 2019.

Kornfield, Jack. *Buddha's Little Instruction Book*. London: Rider, 2018.

Neff, Kristin. *Self-Compassion: The Proven Power of Being Kind to Yourself*. New York: William Morrow, 2015.

Neff, Kristin and Christopher Germer. *The Mindful Self-Compassion Workbook: A Proven Way to Accept Yourself, Build Inner Strength, and Thrive*. New York: Guilford Press, 2018.

Pennebaker, James W. and Joshua M. Smyth. *Opening Up by Writing it Down: How Expressive Writing Improves Health and Eases Emotional Pain*. New York: Guilford Press, 2016.

Rogers, Fred. "2002 Dartmouth College Commencement Speech." Home.Dartmouth.edu /news/2018/03/revisiting-fred-rogers-2002-commencement-address.

Scartt J. R., "Postpartum Depression in Men." *Innovations in Clinical Neuroscience* 16, no. 5–6 (2019): 11–14.

Siegel, Daniel and Tina Jane Bryson. *The Whole-Brain Child*. New York: Random House, 2015.

Stuart, Scott and Michael Robertson. *Interpersonal Psychotherapy: A Clinician's Guide*. London: Hodder Arnold, 2012.

Weir, K. *Nurtured by Nature*. APA.org/monitor/2020/04/nurtured-nature (accessed October 15, 2021).

Woolf, Virginia. *A Room of One's Own*. Oxford: Oxford Paperbacks, 1992.

Acknowledgments

I'm grateful for the support from my husband and children, who encouraged me from the start, when I thought it was a wild idea to write this journal after the most intense 18 months of our lives (COVID).

I want to acknowledge my mother, my role model from day one, who, with three books under her belt, brought her usual cheerleading, enthusiasm, and proofreading skills to the table. Thank you for the encouragement throughout this process and always.

To my colleagues in perinatal mental health, especially Karen Kleiman of the Postpartum Stress Center, where I took the most impactful training of my career; PHA for the ongoing support and case consultation all these years; and PSI—your trainings are so good and always so much fun to attend.

About the Author

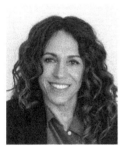

RACHEL RABINOR, LCSW, PMH-C, is a perinatal mental health certified, licensed clinical social worker in San Diego. She specializes in the assessment and treatment of perinatal mood and anxiety disorders and reproductive mental health. She is passionate about helping those struggling with infertility, miscarriage, loss, and birth trauma. Rachel is trained in various evidence-based treatments, including eye movement desensitization and reprocessing (EMDR), interpersonal psychotherapy, and parent-child interaction therapy. She has led postpartum support groups for new mothers and currently offers mind–body infertility groups. Rachel is a member of San Diego's Postpartum Health Alliance and has served on its executive board.

CPSIA information can be obtained
at www.ICGtesting.com
Printed in the USA
JSHW012123210322
24097JS00009B/182

9 781638 783282